Ron Clark, M.D.

SURVIVING THE
EMERGENCY ROOM

Expecting the Unexpected

ISBN: 1450553125
ISBN-13: 9781450553124
Library of Congress Control Number: 2010901248

**For my children.
I love being an emergency physician,
but I love being Daddy more.**

DISCLAIMER

The opinions, advice, and explanations provided in this book are solely those of the author. This book is for informational proposes only and should not substitute for the medical judgment of your physician.

CONTENTS

PREFACE

I have observed over the first few years of my emergency medicine career that patients seeking medical care in the emergency department setting often have misconceptions and misguided expectations. This book is intended to serve as a resource for those that may seek emergency medical care. This essentially includes everyone, as accidents and illness can and will happen to all of us.

The title of this book is actually a misnomer, as the emergency room should more correctly be referred to as the emergency department. This is because in most acute emergency medical care settings, there are many rooms with different functions, and medical care is delivered by many different staff members that function as a unit. At times, this complex medical care delivery system can seem overwhelming.

This book was written with the waiting emergency department patient in mind and with the realization that some may finish this book before their emergency medical care is completed. Each chapter is intended to provide quick, efficient, and enjoyable reading that is relevant to everyone. It explains the emergency medical system so that patients and family members can understand it and use it to their advantage. It will allow you to know where to go, what to ask for, and what to expect. With this knowledge, the healing process can begin.

1
THE BOX OF CHOCOLATES

"LIFE IS LIKE A BOX OF CHOCOLATES. You never know what you're gonna get." This famous Forrest Gump quote can be applied to emergency medical care on many levels. First, medical illness of any type is often initially unknown and unexpected. A patient may not feel well, but may not know or understand the medical problem. It is a scary thought when one realizes that medical illness can strike anyone, anywhere, at anytime, for any reason. The patient has no control over this process and illness often strikes without warning. Illness does not discriminate and strikes randomly. Men, women, the old, and the young are all potential emergency department patients.

Compared with other venues for medical care, patients presenting to the emergency department have to deal with a very different set of conditions. As each emergency department at any given hospital has its own strengths and weaknesses, emergency medical care is truly the box of chocolates. The patient often has little control over the person or type of emergency medical care that is administered.

Most people are unaware of their community emergency medical resources and only find out what is available when they have an emergent medical need. To the patient, emergency medical care is the great unknown. Yet, most people have blind faith that the emergency medical system will be able to take care of them whenever they dial 911. What is important to recognize is that each hospital has different emergency medical resources.

The first variable is the skill level, experience, and qualifications of the emergency physician or physician assistant caring for the patient. Another variable is the fact that the patient is subjected to unfamiliar emergency department nurses and techs, whose own clinical skills are unknown to the patient. There is also great variability in availability of medical and surgical specialists as well as the availability of radiology studies. Each hospital has different types of special procedure equipment, and each emergency department has its own unique layout and physical appearance.

In almost any other medical setting, the patient decides the physician that will take care of them. This is not true with emergency medical care, as the physician on duty is often unknown to the patient and the presenting medical problem is often unexpected. The patient has no time to plan for their medical care so they are forced to take what and whom they get.

As with any other type of medicine, each physician has his or her own strengths and weaknesses. Most patients would hope that their physician is capable of treating their particular medical issue. For the patient in an emergency medical care setting, a better hope would be for the treating physician to be able to recognize their particular medical problem properly. The best emergency physicians are able to recognize symptom patterns and make the proper diagnosis. This is the key to efficient and appropriate emergency medical care. If the emergency physician can treat the medical problem, he or she will. If the emergency physician is unqualified to treat the patient, a specialist will be called. **The key for emergency medical care is, first, to know what you have, and then who can fix it.** The patient has little control over this medical decision process and must hope their emergency physician is capable and qualified.

2

JACK-OF-ALL-TRADES

THE SPECIALTY OF EMERGENCY MEDICINE can be viewed as a shallow "medical ocean," where the emergency physician knows a little bit about everything. An emergency physician has training in virtually all aspects of medicine; he or she should be able to diagnose any potential medical problem, regardless if it is emergent, urgent, or non-urgent. Exclusively, the emergency physician or physician assistant handles most medical conditions, and the majority of patients are discharged from the emergency department. The challenging aspect of emergency medical care is that the emergency physician must be comfortable treating any patient for any imaginable medical problem. There are no limitations, and there is seemly no end to the potential medical problems that may show up in the emergency department. Therefore, the emergency physician must rely on broad and diversified medical training combined with clinical experience to properly care for the different varieties of patients who may seek emergency medical care.

Emergency medicine is based on acute symptom recognition, which then results in a differential diagnosis. The job of the emergency physician is then to order the proper work up, which, in turn, will confirm the correct diagnosis.

The emergency physician will then administer the proper medical treatment. The more training and experience, the easier and more efficient this process becomes.

The difficult patients are the ones that present with vague medical complaints that may result in a broad differential diagnosis. Emergency medical care works best when the emergency physician can focus the medical complaint, which for some patients is next to impossible.

Once the diagnosis is made, the issue then becomes who is able and available to treat the medical problem if it is outside the expertise of the emergency physician. For example, an emergency physician can diagnose a patient with an inflamed appendix, but only a general surgeon can remove the appendix. If you have chest pain, an emergency physician can diagnose a heart attack, but only an interventional cardiologist can open a blocked coronary artery with a balloon.

In short, the emergency physician is required to make the correct diagnosis, but at times may be unable to render the proper medical care. This creates a liability issue where the emergency physician is dependent on other specialists. This dependency can place the emergency physician and the patient in a precarious situation.

3

AN ARMY OF ONE

MOST GOOD EMERGENCY PHYSICIANS know what they can handle, and more importantly, they can recognize when they need a specialist to consult, treat, or admit a patient. Often if a diagnosis is not considered, it will be missed. A good emergency physician must determine, often within a short period of time, when to call in the troops. Hopefully, your emergency physician will not be the general in an army of one.

Specialty medical consultants are physicians with unique knowledge, medical training, technical skill, and experience. They include both medical physicians and surgeons, often with many years of medical training in a particular medical condition or organ system (heart, lungs, digestive system, brain, or any other part of the body that you can think of). A specialty medical consultant is often consulted when the patient has a complicated medical condition or when the patient requires a special procedure that the emergency physician is unable to provide.

The emergency department is open for all patients, but often is unequipped to handle all emergencies. Ask for an expert if one is available, or better yet, call the hospital prior to arrival (if possible) to determine if the hospital has the medical specialty coverage that you may need. This avoids the unnecessary frustration with transfer issues to tertiary (higher level of medical coverage) medical centers, wasted time, and a delay in appropriate medical care.

The tough part in guiding your medical care is that you (or your physician for that matter) may not initially know that you need a specialty medical consultant. It may be shocking to you, but all hospitals are not created equally and most will struggle with making their specialists take call twenty-four hours a day for all seven days of the week. Most hospital emergency departments have a piece of paper at the secretary's desk, which on any given day has blanks, which should be the name of the physician or surgeon on call.

Hopefully, you don't have a massive hand infection if there is no hand surgeon on call or have a severe eye injury if there is no eye doctor on call. Your emergency physician will most likely be angry when he or she realizes that he or she is the unlucky physician who has correctly identified your medical problem but is powerless because the hospital does not have the proper specialty medical consultant available. If your medical problem requires acute surgical intervention, this delay in definitive treatment can lead to a poor outcome. **Poor specialty medical coverage only matters when you are that special patient**.

4

CONTROLLED CHAOS

EMERGENCY MEDICAL CARE AT ITS BASIC LEVEL is about information management. The emergency physician must quickly gather patient data (history, physical exam, responses to previous treatment) and then form a comprehensive medical evaluation and treatment plan. This task may seem relatively easy for the first patient seen. Now multiply this task by the twenty-five or more patients that the physician may be responsible for in a given shift and the task now seems a bit more daunting. Emergency medicine is often likened to drinking out of a fire hose. The physician gets flooded with information and has to take as much in as he or she can.

Now imagine yourself as that twenty-fifth patient. Do you think that your doctor will remember every last detail of your medical issue? The answer to this question is probably no, but your doctor should remember the important points. The take home point is that you should keep your interactions with the physician brief and to the point. Tell the physician the main reason that you came to the emergency department (instead of your regular physician) and quickly review your major symptoms. Giving your physician only the pertinent facts will allow the physician the best chance to focus your medical care. By focusing your medical care, the physician will most likely order the proper studies and render the proper medical treatment.

The emergency department is a kind of controlled chaos. The emergency physician is often managing all ages of patients, with all types of medical and surgical problems, all at the same time. Some physicians will write things down (such as a heart murmur, which eye is red, which part of the body has a laceration, etc.) so that they can remember and keep different patients straight. Don't be offended if the physician is writing while you are talking, this type of organization should be encouraged. Liken this to your shopping list. Would you remember everything you need without it? The difference is instead of milk and eggs, your life may be at stake.

Many patients feel that they need to be excessively social with their physicians and often make small talk (unrelated to their current medical problem). These extra facts and information can often side track your medical care. If you want to be social, go to a dinner party. Remember, your physician is in the information management business. The more water in the "medical hose" for the physician to drink, the greater the chance that an important piece of information may be missed. If this happens, you will both be all wet.

5

THE DANGER ZONE

EMERGENCY DEPARTMENTS ARE RUN SIMILAR to factories with the doctors working in shifts. At most hospitals, there is a day shift, an evening shift, and a night shift. The period of transition time between one doctor's shift and the next is referred to as "sign out." During sign out, one doctor is often tired and wants to leave, and the other is fresh but overwhelmed with the work ahead. During this period of time, the departing emergency physician will "run the board" and go through the name, room, and treatment plan for each patient still in the emergency department. Because most emergency department studies and medical interventions can be done quickly, a single medical provider will treat most patients. At sign out time, these fortunate patients who have had their emergency medical care completed will be either admitted or discharged. The emergency physician receiving sign out will most likely have no interaction with these patients.

Those patients who are left without a final disposition are in medical limbo. This can be due to pending labs, radiology studies, or waiting for a specialist to come to the emergency department. Another reason for a patient to be signed out to the next physician is if that patient is not feeling better. This can be due to inappropriate or inadequate prior medical care, malingering (fabricating medical symptoms for a secondary gain such as pain medication or time off from work), or the possibility that the patient actually has something serious. It is often difficult for the emergency physician receiving sign out to paint the correct medical picture quickly. For this reason, most emergency physicians prefer to keep patient sign outs to a minimum so that the medical canvas does not get too complicated.

Most emergency physicians like to evaluate and treat patients by themselves. They often do not like receiving sign out on patients who have been treated by someone else. This is because the previous medical evaluation and plan may lead them down the wrong path. This sign out time can potentially bias the emergency physician and place the patient in danger. For example, the emergency physician going home may tell the physician receiving sign out that a patient with a headache simply has a migraine and can be discharged when he or she feels better. In reality, this patient might have meningitis or a brain bleed. These are two "can't miss" diagnoses that need a spinal tap and a head CT scan, respectively. If the emergency physician does not consider the diagnosis, the diagnosis can easily be missed. The take home point is that in each medical interaction with a different physician, the patient should make sure that the physician currently providing medical treatment is aware of all the symptoms and has reviewed all the medical studies that were done.

Sometimes a new physician's perspective can pick out something that was missed. Other times, a new physician can make the medical management water murkier. Be aware of this sign out time and if you have a sense that your medical care is going to take a good chunk of time, ask your physician when his or her shift ends and request that your physician say "good-bye" at the end of the shift. Request that your new physician and your departing physician come into your room together during this "good-bye" time. While both of your doctors are in the room, request that your medical care to this point be reviewed so that everyone is on the same page, but beware…you have just entered **The Danger Zone**.

Patients need to be aware that the danger zone is most risky for the patient during the nighttime.

6

ON THE NIGHT TRAIN

THE NIGHT SHIFT AT MOST EMERGENCY DEPARTMENTS
is a totally different practice environment than during the
day. As the patient census goes down at night, most hospitals schedule less emergency department staff. A typical
busy community hospital may have three day-shift physicians and three evening-shift physicians, but usually only one
night-shift physician. This means that all active medical problems in the emergency department ultimately become the
responsibility of a single night physician.

It only takes one very critically ill patient to clog up the
entire night operation. For example, if a patient has a cardiac arrest, the emergency physician who is "running the
code" will be actively directing the resuscitation and performing any invasive procedures that may be needed. This
critical care time may take minutes to hours depending on
the unique medical needs of the patient. When the emergency physician is finished, he or she may find that there are
many other very sick patients that have been waiting without proper medical attention. Because there is only one
emergency physician, there is no one else to call. The only
saving grace is that some emergency departments employ a
physician assistant to help care for patients during the night

shift. These physician assistants are often very experienced and can be extremely helpful to make the emergency medical management of patients more efficient.

The limited medical staff issue is then further complicated by the limited availability of radiology studies. Some emergency departments have limited availability of CT scans, MRIs, and Ultrasound during the night. As with the specialty medical consultants that were detailed in a previous chapter, the availability of these special radiology studies only matters if you are that special patient that needs them quickly to address your acute medical issue. If the study is emergently needed and unavailable, the patient will have to be transferred to another hospital. This transfer process can be an annoying experience for both the night shift physician and the patient, with both wishing that it were daytime.

Often, there is limited availability of ancillary service providers during the night. For example, a patient and family may have to wait until morning for a social worker to be available to place a patient at a nursing home. If a patient is in the emergency department for a psychiatric issue, they may have to wait until morning to be assessed by the crisis intervention team. These types of patients are commonly referred to as "hold overs." In general, the patients who are waiting until morning for a particular social issue to be addressed are very easy to care for and the night shift physician will have limited contact. In contrast, if the patient is waiting in the emergency department for definitive care for an acute psychotic episode, the emergency physician's night just got a bit more colorful, as you will see in the next chapter.

7

THE CRISIS PATIENT: MAKING THE VOICES WORK FOR YOU

THE EMERGENCY DEPARTMENT IS OFTEN THE END of the road for the crisis patient. These patients often have substance abuse issues or mental illness. Many of these patients are classified as dual diagnosis, where they have mental illness compounded with alcohol or drug dependence. Other crisis patients may present to the emergency department with no history of mental illness, but may be depressed, anxious, suicidal, or homicidal after a life-altering event, such as the death of a loved one. In general, patients who are in crisis usually find their way to one of two places: jail or the emergency department.

Often times, law enforcement will be called to the scene of a person who is acting strangely. The person may be walking in the middle of a busy street, may be nude in public, may be talking to him or herself, and often times may look very disheveled. The police officer at the scene has the difficult job of quickly determining, first, if the patient is dangerous or not and, second, hopefully considering if the patient has a medical condition that needs care. If it seems that the patient may need medical care, emergency medical services will be called for a medical assessment at the scene and transportation (sometimes handcuffed) to the emergency department.

Emergency medical services will often radio ahead to the emergency department that a potential crisis patient is about to arrive. This gives the emergency department a chance to prepare. A good emergency department staff will hope for the best, but expect the worst. Hospital security will be notified to stand by in case the patient is violent and requires physical restraint. Depending on the local medical protocols, the emergency physician may have already given the emergency medical service providers permission to sedate the patient in the ambulance. If not, the emergency nurse may be standing by with intramuscular injection medications to be used if the need arises.

When the crisis patient arrives, the emergency physician will quickly assess patient and staff safety, rule out underlying medical conditions, and then finally treat mental illness, if it exists. First, the emergency physician will evaluate if the patient is a danger to him or herself or others (including emergency department staff). If the patient is deemed a threat and escalation of the situation is likely, the emergency physician has three options for de-escalation: verbal, chemical, and physical.

A good emergency physician, first, will verbally try to reassure the patient that they are safe and will often allow the patient to vent their feelings. Clear limits will be set from this first medical interaction and the patient will be told what needs to happen. If cooperative, the patient will be undressed to make sure there are no weapons, drugs or other things that may injure the patient or a staff member.

If the emergency physician is unsuccessful in trying to calm the patient, he or she may tell the patient to take a pill to try to calm him or her down. If the patient refuses, the emergency physician may be forced to give a sedative medication involuntarily to the patient using an intramuscular injection. If a patient is deemed a threat to him or herself or others, the emergency physician has the mandated right and duty to provide medical care, as the patient can be considered incompetent to refuse care. Competency is a legal term, but in the trenches of acute emergency medical care, as long as the emergency physician is working in the best interests of the patient and doing so safely, the medical care administered would most likely be viewed as appropriate if questioned.

If the chemical restraint does not work to control the patient, then physical restraint using four-point restraints will be ordered. Both of the patient's arms and legs will be strapped to the bed. This requires a trained team of security personnel with the proper equipment available and is the main reason why security is called to the room for any potentially violent crisis patient.

The goal of crisis de-escalation is to use the least amount of force when caring for crisis patients. The ideal succession of verbal reassurance, followed by chemical sedation, and only then physical restraint, is at times, impossible. A patient, who is violent, thrashing on the stretcher, swearing, and spitting, may already be restrained with handcuffs or other means prior to emergency department arrival. Crisis patients can be unpredictable, and at times their emotions may explode, which may require security personnel to restrain them physically while the nurse gets the intramuscular injection medications. A good emergency physician will know to medicate the crisis patient in a prophylactic manner so that violence is kept to a minimum.

After the emergency physician has assured the safety of the patient and the emergency department staff, the emergency physician's next duty is to determine rapidly if there is a medical problem that is causing the patient's altered mental status. An experienced emergency physician knows that medical disease comes in many different forms and that if not considered, a medical disease may be missed. Therefore, there are some basic things that are done with any patient who is acting confused, disoriented, or inappropriate.

The emergency physician will order basic blood work to exclude electrolyte imbalances, including high or low blood sugar. For any potential crisis patient, a blood toxicology analysis for the presence of alcohol, Tylenol, and aspirin should be sent. As these three substances are readily available to the public, crisis patients have the opportunity to take them in quantities that may be lethal. The emergency physician will also check for mind-altering illegal substances such as cocaine, amphetamines, marijuana, and opiates. A prudent emergency physician will check these things on every crisis patient, as some crisis patients will not disclose that these substances were taken. The emergency physician should trust, but verify.

During this medical clearance process, the emergency physician may order a head CT scan to see if there is a stroke, trauma, or bleeding process. Under certain clinical situations, the emergency physician may also want other additional radiology studies to exclude physical injury.

Once the patient is medically cleared, the final task is to evaluate and then treat mental illness if it exists. The difficulty with emergency medicine is that the emergency physician only has a brief "snap shot" of the patient's behavior in the emergency room. Therefore, the emergency physician must rely on others, including police, emergency medical services, family, and friends, to paint an accurate medical picture. Sometimes, a patient who is combative at the scene may be quiet in the emergency department. The emergency physician has the difficult task of determining who is at immediate risk.

If the patient is brought to the emergency department by law enforcement, most states have a police emergency evaluation request form that is completed. This form should be detailed and specific as to the patient's inappropriate actions or statements so that their behavior is properly documented. The same is true if you are a loved one of a patient with mental illness. If you bring a patient with mental illness to the emergency department, request that your concerns be documented in the medical record by either the physician or nurse. As some patients with mental illness are not aware that they have a problem, detailed accounts of behavior, statements, and actions will allow the emergency physician the best chance to make the right medical decision. As emergency physicians work in shifts, it is important that your concerns are written down so that they are not lost or forgotten during staff changes.

If the emergency physician feels that the crisis patient does not have an acute psychiatric problem that needs hospitalization and is not a danger to him or herself or others, the patient will most likely be discharged. If the patient is deemed to have an acute psychiatric condition that requires hospitalization, the patient will be admitted to the hospital or transferred to another hospital that has in-patient psychiatric facilities.

Patients who have mental illness, and their family members, should be aware that many hospitals do not have in-patient psychiatric services. **Therefore, if there is a strong indication that you or your loved one will need to be admitted, go to a hospital that has in-patient psychiatric beds to avoid the need for hospital transfer**. If you or your loved one has a psychiatrist with hospital admitting privileges, go to the hospital where they can admit you. Sometimes, it is possible to request that your psychiatrist directly admit you to the hospital, thereby avoiding the emergency department entirely.

For guardians who have a younger patient with mental illness, call ahead to the emergency department to see if the hospital has pediatric in-patient psychiatric services. This will avoid transfer issues and lengthy emergency department stays, as most states have a very limited number of in-patient pediatric psychiatric beds. If you take your child to an emergency department that has pediatric psychiatric resources, you can most likely avoid the frustrating transfer process.

Try to choose a hospital that is close to home, so that if the patient wants visits from family or friends, people can visit your loved one to show support for them. Mental illness is often a lonely road and family involvement and support can often be the difference between treatment success and failure.

If the patient is a danger to him or herself or others and needs admission, they cannot refuse care. In this situation, the emergency physician can "paper" the patient. This process, known as a physician emergency certificate, can involuntarily commit a patient to the hospital. Most states have a maximum number of committal days for the initial certificate. If the patient is in the hospital longer, the patient has the right to have a hearing with a judge to determine if the committal needs to be extended.

Due to limited hospital resources, sometimes there is disagreement between the emergency physician and the patient or family member as to when the patient should be discharged from the hospital. Many emergency physicians will request that a family member or friend sign the patient out of the emergency department. This allows the emergency physician to document that someone else is aware of the discharged patient and assumes that this patient will have support.

If the emergency department wants to discharge your loved one and you truly feel the patient is dangerous, do not voluntarily come to the emergency department and sign the patient out. This forces the emergency physician to take complete responsibility for the patient should there be an immediate problem after discharge. Another option is to request that the emergency nurse document your particular concerns, as this will force the emergency physician to address them. Most physicians are risk averse and will take the necessary steps to avoid medical-legal liability. In the end, the emergency physician wants to do the right thing.

Good emergency physicians have thick skin. They do not get rattled by insults and are not scared to care for those that are deemed undesirable by others. Whether the patient is intoxicated or has mental illness, or both, most crisis patients do have a legitimate medical problem. It is the duty of the emergency physician to provide medical care. The emergency physician is there to advocate and protect those who are unable to care for themselves. Most emergency physicians view their medical management of vulnerable, compromised, and difficult crisis patients as just a part of the job of being on the front lines of medicine.

Most people rest assured knowing that their local emergency department is there to care for these patients that everyone knows about, but few speak of.

8

KNOW WHAT CAN KILL YOU

KNOW WHAT CAN KILL YOU. You should know your medical problems, surgeries, medications, and allergies, otherwise you are just a black box, and that can be dangerous. Many times the emergency physician must order very powerful medications to make you better. The trade off is that there is always a risk of drug interactions and side effects when medications are given. To minimize potential complications, you should always be honest with your physician and responsible enough to remember (or write down) your basic medical information. A written sheet with your personal medical and surgical history, medications with dosages, and your doctor and pharmacy phone numbers should always be kept in your wallet or purse. For those with serious medical conditions, such as diabetes, heart disease, or seizure disorders, a medical alert bracelet is recommended. These bracelets can often give important medical clues to the paramedic or emergency physician if you are unresponsive. It is also important that you carry your loved ones emergency contact information with you. In an emergency medical situation, emergency physicians often look to family members and friends for important medical information that may guide or alter emergency medical care. If you or a loved one is experiencing an emergent medical problem and there is no time to write all your medications down on paper, simply bring the medicine bottles with you. The emergency physician will then know the medication with its proper dose and the pharmacy phone number so that other medications can be determined and dosages confirmed.

Patients often unrealistically expect the emergency physician to know everything about them from the moment they step foot in the room. Often times, there is a delay in obtaining old medical records, so the emergency physician must rely on the patient to paint an accurate picture of his or her medical problems. It is also prudent for any physician to ask the patient directly about medical problems, as information often changes from the previous medical record.

People's lives are always in a dynamic state of change. Physicians should ask about current medical problems, medications, and allergies. There is less likelihood that a mistake will be made when the information given is accurate and verified. To an emergency physician, a new patient is a complete stranger. Often times, the patient will get upset when asked the same questions by the nurse and then the doctor. It is important to remember that each medical interaction with a different provider is a new encounter.

Most medical providers operate on the assumption that they must personally verify certain information for themselves. A physician may ask the patient for a complete list of all their medications, including herbal and over-the-counter medications. Many of the powerful medications used in the emergency department have known drug interactions. The experienced emergency physician will want to confirm medication safety prior to ordering a medication. The physician may also want to confirm a patient's medication dosage so the patient is not overmedicated. When a medication is ordered, the nurse will not give the medication without asking the patient about allergies. An adverse reaction associated with improper medication administration is one of the most common mistakes made when rendering emergency medical care. Emergency nurses are keenly aware of this fact and will verbally confirm the patient's allergy status each and every time a medication is administered.

Remember that safety in the medical field starts with the responsible patient and ends with the competent physician and nurse.

9

TURNING WEAKNESS INTO STRENGTH

MANY OF THE PATIENTS THAT USE the emergency department are there because of a particular medical condition. These medical problems often require special interventions in a timely manner. You should make the most of your medical problems and use them to your advantage. For example if you are a diabetic and you are hungry, tell the nurse or doctor that you need to eat or your sugar may drop. The doctor will see to it that you eat as long as you do not require an intervention that needs sedation. If you are a potential surgical candidate, your doctor will not let you eat.

If you have a history of migraine headaches, ask for a quiet room and for the lights to be off if that helps your headache. If you have a fracture, ask for additional pain medication if you need it. If you have a heart condition, inform the nurse or physician immediately when being triaged so that an appropriate room with a cardiac monitor can be arranged. If you have a lung problem and are short of breath, ask for a breathing treatment and some oxygen. Because the oxygen is often connected to the wall in a room, this request may get you into a room faster.

Remember to speak up and advocate for yourself or a loved one, as this is the best way for you to obtain the best care for your particular medical condition. However, when making special requests, you need to be aware that you may become the squeaky wheel.

10

THE SQUEAKY WHEEL

THE EMERGENCY DEPARTMENT IS OFTEN an extremely busy place. Doctors and nurses juggle multiple patients at the same time. Many of these patients have complicated medical requirements that need to be addressed. As health-care providers are human beings, they can only be in one place at a time. This fact often results in patients feeling like they had very little "face time" with their medical providers. This leaves patients feeling dissatisfied and, at times, angry. Some patients will continually push the call button to bring the nurse into the room, or they will repeatedly demand to speak with the physician. Some patients are nice about making requests and others are not.

As the number of special requests increases, the patient starts to transform into the squeaky wheel. The key to becoming an effective squeaky wheel is to realize that you need to pick your battles. If the nurse is in your room, ask for an additional blanket, food, or medical update at that time. Don't let the nurse leave without your concerns being addressed. This is the time to speak up, as this is your personal face time. Remember once the nurse or doctor leaves your room, the face time is shifted to someone else.

Write down questions for the nurse or the doctor so that your face time is used efficiently.

Be aware that being overly demanding or excessively calling for the nurse or doctor can often be met with unintended consequences. The nurse or doctor may consciously or subconsciously label you as a difficult patient and avoid your room or your side of the hallway. This may result in a lack of medical reassessment, which can be a recipe for disaster in emergency medical care.

As emergency medical providers have multiple tasks to complete in a short period of time, they often take the path of least resistance. If you are becoming the point of resistance, your medical care may be adversely affected. Your medical provider may subconsciously minimize your medical complaints and that can lead to a delay or failure to obtain the correct diagnosis. In medicine, as in life, perception is everything.

The key to being a successful squeaky wheel is to speak up and advocate without being rude. Medical providers are people with feelings and emotions. Acknowledge to the medical provider that you realize they are busy and thank them for addressing your particular concern. Being polite and expressing a small amount of gratitude will go a long way with an emergency nurse or physician that is often not thanked properly. In this case, the doctor or nurse may go out of their way to make sure that the "nice" squeaky wheel receives quick and efficient medical care.

Remember the squeaky wheel gets the grease, but unfortunately, if the wheel gets too slick, the patient ends up being run over.

11

NO ROOM AT THE INN

IN BUSY EMERGENCY DEPARTMENTS with limited space, patients are often seen and examined in the hallway. The physician may do a quick cursory physical examination that may miss a potential medical problem. If the patient is not undressed because of being in the hallway, the physician may miss a rash that may be contagious or leg swelling that may mean there is a blood clot. The emergency physician has the responsibility to treat the entire patient and missing a diagnosis because of where the patient's stretcher is located is unacceptable.

So what can the unlucky and embarrassed patient do while hoards of people are walking by? First, tell the nurse that you are uncomfortable in the hallway and if there are no rooms available, ask to be placed in a quiet section of the hallway where there is less foot traffic. Second, when the emergency physician finally comes to examine you, ask if you can be examined in a room so that nothing is missed. Most emergency physicians will agree to this reasonable request and will simply move someone else out of a room, especially if they have already been examined and are just waiting for test results. Now you have the room for the time being.

The issue of emergency department overcrowding is a national problem. Most hospitals do not have adequate space to send patients immediately up to the floor after an admission decision has been made. The reasons for this are complex, but it essentially comes down to supply and demand. The supply of hospital beds is relatively low and the demand for these beds is high, as more patients are using emergency medical services each day.

Emergency department patients who are waiting for an in-patient hospital bed are commonly known as "boarders." These patients often get stuck in limbo as they wait for a patient from the floor to be discharged so that they can have the bed. To make matters worse, some patients have special needs such as needing to be on a cardiac monitor or needing to be isolated due to a potential infectious disease. These patients can often linger in the emergency department for days before appropriate in-patient accommodations can be made.

If the delay to obtain a bed starts to become unbearable, ask the emergency nurse for an update. Ask if the delay is due to a lack of a bed or a lack of admitting medical orders. If the delay is due to a bed shortage, you are stuck, and unless the hospital can open additional floors, expect a prolonged emergency department stay. If the issue is a lack of medical orders, request to speak with the admitting doctor. It is often possible for the doctor to write the admitting orders first and do the rest of the paperwork later so that you can get out the emergency department in a timely manner. Another option would be to ask if the emergency physician would be willing to write "holding orders" for the admitting doctor so that the patient can get to the floor faster.

Remember the complexities of a hospital system are similar to the airline industry—expect delays.

12

THE GOOD, THE BAD, AND THE UGLY

ONCE THE EMERGENCY PHYSICIAN DECIDES to admit a patient, medical management is then transferred to either the patient's personal physician or a hospitalist physician. The patient's personal physician or a designated hospitalist physician will evaluate the patient in the emergency department to determine his or her medical needs and to coordinate the in-patient medical care plan. Many primary care doctors are increasingly choosing not to care for their patients in the hospital. If your primary care physician does not provide in-patient medical care at the hospital, the hospitalist physician will then become your doctor during your hospital stay.

A hospitalist physician is usually a primary care doctor who is paid by the hospital to provide medical care for patients when they are admitted into the hospital. These patients are referred to as unassigned patients, as they either have no primary care physician or their private physician does not have admitting privileges at the hospital where they are now admitted. These physicians coordinate all aspects of in-patient medical care including medication management, performing medical procedures, and obtaining specialty consultations. Increasing numbers of busy primary care doctors are using the hospitalist service to manage their admitted patients. There are advantages and disadvantages to this relatively new medical arrangement.

The good news for a patient being managed by a hospitalist physician is that this doctor's career is dedicated to quality, efficient in-patient medical care. This physician has intimate knowledge of the hospital system and is usually able to get things done in an efficient manner. The hospitalist physician knows who to call for special procedures and usually has a good working relationship with the nursing staff. When new medical problems arise or the patient's medical condition changes, the hospitalist physician is physically there to provide direct patient care. This is in contrast to the medical care of a private admitting physician, who may be at the office and unable to render direct medical care when needed.

The bad news is that the hospitalist physician is not the patient's regular doctor, and for some patients this arrangement can be impersonal. The patient is a complete stranger to the hospitalist physician, and medical care has to start with the basics. The patient must review all their medical problems, medications, allergies, and social situations with this new physician. The patient's own personal physician would have already known these things. As with any medical interaction, there is a trust issue. The temporary nature of the hospitalist medical service makes building trust difficult for some patients. Trust takes time to develop and many patients do not feel a bond with their hospitalist physician. Unfortunately, many in-patient medical interactions are brief and patient stays are short, which results in poor medical bonding. You should know if your own doctor uses the hospitalist service prior to going to the hospital. This will avoid the shock of being cared for by an unfamiliar face.

A lack of communication can create an ugly situation for the hospitalist patient. Communication is the key to proper medical care, and lack of it is when medical mistakes can be made. The patient may not feel comfortable with the hospitalist physician and this may cause the patient to limit the medical information that he or she discloses. Patients may have substance abuse issues, sexually transmitted diseases, or other personal issues that they do not want an unfamiliar doctor to know about. These types of medical problems, at times, can lead to future in-patient medical complications. For example, an undisclosed alcoholic may have an alcohol withdrawal seizure in the hospital because of not drinking alcohol. If the hospitalist physician is made aware of these types of medical issues in advance, medications can be given to avoid complications.

Some private physicians can abuse their arrangement with the hospitalist service. As they are not responsible for providing medical care once the patient enters the hospital, they can be quick to send patients to the emergency department for difficult or annoying patients that they do not want to deal with at the office. The private doctor knows that the emergency physician will render emergency medical care and if the patient needs to be admitted, the hospitalist physician will medically manage the patient. The private doctor is effectively out of the medical loop, as they can hand off any patient, for any reason, at any time. This medical arrangement creates the potential for abuse.

The overworked hospitalist service is essentially doing the work that was previously done by private doctors. As previously stated, communication is the key to excellent medical care. Difficulty arises when some of these private physicians do not want to be bothered or contacted. This is particularly the case at night, when some private physicians will not return answering service pages to the hospital. This is because they know that there are capable doctors at the hospital, and they do not feel responsibility for any aspect of hospital care. This passing of the "medical buck" is unfortunate, but at times, true.

The transfer of medical responsibility from the private physician to the hospitalist physician has one final ugly consequence. As the hospitalist physician is only responsible for hospital care, there is often pressure not to admit patients when the medical service is busy or the hospital is full. This can cause the hospitalist physician to block an admission if the patient is on the "medical fence." Most emergency physicians are conservative in their medical care and if medical admission is considered, it should be done. Many of these blocked admissions should stay to be observed and properly cared for. When a patient is discharged from the emergency department only to return a short while later, the patient is commonly labeled a "bounce back."

13
THE BLESSING IN DISGUISE

EMERGENCY PHYSICIANS USE THE TERM bounce back to describe a patient who decides to return to the emergency department after he or she has recently been seen. Some physicians dread these bounce back patients, as it often implies that they were dissatisfied with their medical care or their medical condition deteriorated. Most emergency physicians will get a pit in their stomach when a colleague notifies them that their emergency department patient returned for additional medical care. Some physicians get angry or feel embarrassed when a patient returns back to the same emergency department from which he or she was just discharged. Although these feelings of inadequacy are normal emotions, these particular bounce back patients can often be a blessing in disguise.

The fact that the bounce back patient returned back to the emergency department requesting medical care implies that the patient is alive. Emergency medicine is like any other medical specialty, and serious illnesses can be misdiagnosed and mismanaged. Unfortunately for the emergency physician, there is often very little follow up on patients who have been discharged from the emergency department, as the emergency physician will likely never see them again. If the patient does return to the emergency department, being alive is much better than being dead, as the emergency physician has a second chance to render the proper medical care if something was previously missed.

If you feel that you or a loved one received inadequate medical care, it is perfectly appropriate to return back to the same emergency department or seek an emergent second opinion at another hospital. Some diseases present atypically and clinical signs and symptoms may have changed by the time you return to seek additional medical care. A good emergency physician will always welcome you to return to the emergency department, at any time, if your symptoms persist or worsen. If you decide to return to the emergency department, this second medical look may be from a different perspective. Often, a missed medical diagnosis can be corrected if the initial physician or a colleague is afforded a second glance. **Don't be too stubborn or proud to deny a physician the opportunity to re-examine you if you feel something was missed**. This second chance can be a blessing for both of you.

14

NOT ROCKET SCIENCE

EMERGENCY MEDICAL CARE IS A TEAM EFFORT with both the physician and the patient playing on the same team. There are certain common sense responsibilities for the physician and another set for the patient. Poor medical care is often the result of deviation from common sense principles.

One of the most important skills of an emergency physician is symptom recognition. Once a certain set of symptoms are identified, the proper tests can be ordered and an accurate diagnosis can be made. Emergency medicine is not rocket science. The emergency physician needs to have enough knowledge to ask the right questions, and most of the time, this will lead to the correct answer or diagnosis. If the emergency physician were unsure of the correct diagnosis or treatment plan, common sense would dictate that the physician should ask someone else for help.

We should all hope that an emergency physician is not too proud to ask for help. Most emergency physicians have other resources to assist in medical care. During any given shift, most emergency physicians have another emergency physician colleague that is working side by side with them. This colleague may be asked to take a second look at an x-ray or a patient's physical finding. Emergency physicians often "run" a particular medication or treatment option by a colleague when the patient has a complicated medical condition or an uncommon medical disease. This is so the emergency physician does not make a mistake in care. This is similar to a carpenter's "measure twice but cut once" principle.

An emergency physician also has the option of consulting a specialist if the patient has a complicated medical condition, or if he or she requires a medical intervention that the emergency physician is uncomfortable or unqualified to provide. Common sense would dictate that the emergency physician should not perform any medical procedures that are outside the scope of the emergency physician's medical training. If you or a loved one are about to have a medical procedure, ask the physician how many times he or she has performed that particular procedure. If your physician is uncomfortable, you should be too.

Emergency physicians should not be rude or arrogant. All physicians realize that medical illness, at times, is not black and white. This gray zone is particularly true with emergency medical care, and there is a strong possibility that some medical diseases will be missed or treated inappropriately. A good emergency physician will recognize this possibility and try to form trust and a bond with each and every patient. Being kind does not avoid lawsuits, but it does improve the patient's perception of medical care.

A final common sense principle for the emergency physician is not to make assumptions about patients. Physicians who are biased by emotional feelings or who prejudge a patient will often not consider a complete differential diagnosis. This can lead to disaster. For example, the physician who simply thinks that the unresponsive "frequent flyer" alcoholic is simply drunk again, may miss the patient's brain bleed until it is too late.

The label "drug seeker" is a term used by emergency medical care providers for patients who are perceived to be abusing pain medications or who are seeking a pain medication without a legitimate medical problem. Although this perception, at times, is well founded, this term should be avoided. Some of these patients do have chronically painful and debilitating medical problems. More importantly, some of these patients may have serious medical problems that require acute medical intervention. For example, the patient who presents multiple times for low back pain may have an expanding abdominal aortic aneurysm or leak that could potentially kill the patient. This is a "can't miss" diagnosis that is easily missed when inappropriate labels are applied.

Patients should be aware that emergency medical care is a two way street and the patient also has some responsibilities. Common sense would dictate that patients should be open and honest with their physician. Emergency medicine is based on information management, and if the information given is not accurate or complete, medical mistakes can be made.

Patients should realize that the emergency room is not the candy shop. There are some patients who present to the emergency room for medications, particularly for pain, that their primary care doctor is unwilling to provide. This places the emergency physician in the unfair situation of wanting to do the right thing to make the patient comfortable, but not having all the facts to make a prudent decision. There may be a very good reason why the patient's own physician does not want to prescribe a particular medication. There may be side effects, drug interactions with other medications the patient is taking, or the patient may be abusing a particular medication. If your own physician, who knows you best, is not comfortable with a medication, don't take it.

Common sense would dictate that, if possible, you should choose to go to the hospital where your doctor has privileges and where your medical records are kept (EKGs, operative reports, etc.). Most physicians do not like surprises if they can be avoided. For example if you recently had surgery and feel that you are experiencing a complication, go back to the hospital where the surgery was done. For the emergency physician, it is hard to "sell" a patient with a potential surgical complication to a general surgeon that was not the one to do the original surgery and most will request transfer to the original surgeon's hospital to clean up the mess.

Patients should be aware that maloccurrence is not the same as malpractice. Maloccurrence is a less-than-ideal medical outcome. This may be due to expected disease progression or may be a result of a complication from a medication or procedure that was performed. Patients should be aware that not everyone gets better. Those who present to the emergency department with serious emergent medical conditions are already sick, and most medical interventions have inherent risks.

You should expect, and your physician should provide, the risks, benefits, and alternatives to the medical treatment options that are available to you or a loved one. **If you do not understand these options, speak up and ask**

questions. It's your body, ask as many questions as you want until you are comfortable. Asking questions does not hurt, but receiving poor medical care often does.

The final common sense principle for the patient goes back to assumptions. Some patients make unfounded assumptions about their medical providers with no facts to support their feelings. You should not make assumptions about your physician or physician assistant's qualifications or you may make an inappropriate medical request. In other words, be careful what you wish for.

15

BE CAREFUL WHAT YOU WISH FOR

SOME PATIENTS THAT PRESENT TO THE EMERGENCY DEPARTMENT may make inappropriate demands that they may regret. Because most patients do not understand the structure of the emergency medical care system, they may think that what they are requesting may be in their best interests, but that may not always be the case. For example, a patient presenting to the emergency department with a facial laceration may not want the emergency physician to suture it and may instead demand that a plastic surgeon fix it in the emergency department. This demand is made with the assumption that an attending surgeon, who has already completed residency, will be the one to come in. In acute emergency medical care situations of non-life threatening injuries, the attending physician or surgeon will usually be at the office or at home and the person who actually comes to the emergency department to do the "surgical consult" will usually be a resident or physician assistant. The resident or physician assistant will usually call the attending surgeon on the phone, but in most cases, the resident or physician assistant will be the one to render medical care in the emergency department.

As medical care providers have varying levels of skill and ability, the patient who is demanding a surgical consult may be declining the skills of an experienced and capable emergency physician to settle for a first year surgical resident one month out of medical school. This medical provider is called doctor, but may have very little experience, as they are learning on the job. Patients should realize that experience is more important than job title.

Most people probably would not want to fly on a plane with a pilot with one month of experience, yet in emergency medical situations, many patients inadvertently and unknowingly demand the inexperienced. A better strategy for the patient who needs a medical or surgical procedure would be for the patient simply to ask the attending emergency physician about his or her experience. Most emergency physicians would not be offended as this is a valid question. If the emergency physician is experienced and comfortable with the procedure, the emergency physician should do it. If the emergency physician feels that a medical or surgical consult is indicated, a specialist will be called to the emergency department. Patients should be aware to confirm the experience level of the specialist prior to consenting for treatment.

Be careful what you wish for, and remember, making unfounded demands can make you crash and burn.

16
LEARNING ON THE JOB

EMERGENCY MEDICAL CARE IS MOST OFTEN provided by either an academic teaching medical center or by a community hospital. In general, teaching medical centers are usually larger institutions with many different residency or fellowship programs. Residents are doctors who have completed medical school and who are currently training and learning in a given medical or surgical specialty. Over time, these residents gain knowledge and skills that enable them to become competent attending physicians or surgeons, once they graduate from their chosen program. There are some residents who choose to become fellows, where they further their education and training into a subspecialty medical or surgical field. The term "attending" designates a doctor at the end of the "medical education road."

Some community hospitals only have attending physicians and surgeons. Other community hospitals have a mix of attending physicians and residents or fellows. You should be aware that each hospital or medical center has its own unique spectrum of medical providers. If a particular hospital does not support residency or fellowship programs, they usually employ physician assistants to aid the attending physicians and surgeons with rendering medical care.

There are some benefits to being a patient at an academic medical center that trains residents and fellows. Many of these academic medical centers have the most up-to-date and cutting edge medical research and equipment. They may be able to provide medical and surgical treatment options that are unavailable at other hospitals. The trade off is that sometimes the newest medical and surgical techniques are unproven, and the patient can become the guinea pig. The patient can also become the guinea pig for a resident or fellow that is learning a new procedure. As stated in an earlier chapter, experience counts. Residents and fellows are by definition still in medical training, and the patient needs to be aware that an attending physician or surgeon should properly supervise them.

Academic medical centers are often referred to as tertiary medical care centers. They are able to provide a higher level of medical and surgical care because they have medical and surgical specialists that are unavailable at other hospitals. An emergency physician working at an academic medical center often has the luxury of advanced emergency cardiac care for patients with heart attacks, advanced interventional radiology technology and neurology care for patients with strokes, and advanced specialty surgical staff and equipment for patients who have major trauma. When a patient is lucky enough to arrive at an emergency department that has one of these advanced medical or surgical specialists, the emergency physician can simply call the specialist down to the emergency department for a consult. For the patient with an advanced emergent medical or surgical issue that needs specialty care, this is the best place to be as it avoids a delay in definitive emergency medical care.

Residents and fellows are often taught: time is heart muscle or brain tissue. Most attending emergency physicians work outside of academic medical centers and are very aware that a delay in definitive medical care can be disastrous for the patient. The clock is started from the second the patient arrives in the emergency department, and when the emergency physician determines that there is a need for tertiary advanced medical or surgical care, the transfer process begins.

17

THE DREADED TRANSFER

THERE ARE THREE PEOPLE INVOLVED during a hospital-to-hospital transfer. These people include the patient, the transferring physician, and the accepting physician. In general, the physicians on both ends of the phone call dread the hospital transfer process. The patient, also known in this chapter as the "hot potato," is simply caught in the crossfire. The term hot potato is used not to make light of a serious medical emergency, but rather to depict the emotional nature and urgency with which the physician needs to act.

The battle starts when the emergency physician realizes that the resources needed to care for the patient's affliction properly are unavailable at the current facility. Now the emergency physician is holding the hot potato and needs to get rid of it. In general, at this point in time, the physician makes an unsolicited phone call to another equally busy and stressed out physician to take the hot potato off his or her hands. The transferring physician quickly pleads his case, but at this point in the battle, the accepting physician has all the tanks lined up on his or her side.

As the accepting physician is the one who is being solicited, he or she has the fortune of having the coveted resource that the other physician needs. If he or she were the one treating this particular hot potato, he or she would simply make a phone call and admit the patient into his or her hospital. As the transferring physician does not have this luxury, he or she is essentially forced to beg the accepting physician to take the hot potato off his or her hands. As hot potatoes often have complicated medical conditions that necessitate transfer in the first place, the accepting physician already knows that his or her work shift will get a lot busier if he or she says yes.

There are a few things that have to happen in order for the accepting physician to say yes. First, the physician has to take the phone call. As easy as this sounds, the transferring physician is often stuck on hold for a seeming endless period of time waiting for the accepting physician to answer the call. This is because the accepting physician, often times, has his or her own emergent medical problems at his or her facility that are requiring immediate attention, so there is no time to answer the phone.

When the accepting physician has finally been reached, there are a few options. If the accepting emergency physician has the knowledge and skill to treat the hot potato, he or she can say yes, and the transferring physician simply puts that doctor's name on the transfer form. The hot potato is then shipped out of the transferring emergency department with the urgency of a ticking time bomb.

The important aspect to a proper emergency transfer is that the transferring physician must have an accepting physician's name in order to transfer the hot potato. This is because there are anti-dumping laws in the United States so that physicians do not drop their medical problems on other physicians without their knowledge or consent.

If the accepting physician does not personally have the coveted medical skill to treat the hot potato, he or she cannot say yes without conferring with his or her specialist. Now the battle has become more complicated as another physician has been added to the battlefield. The accepting physician is now in the position of using valuable clinical time to first call and then to wait for the specialist to call back. If the specialist says yes, then the hot potato is sent. If the specialist says no, then the transferring physician must call another hospital and start the whole process over.

The specialist may say no for a number of reasons. He or she may not have the proper skill and experience to treat the hot potato. The specialist may not have the time to emergently treat the hot potato especially if he or she already has an emergency that he or she is dealing with. Another reason would be if the specialist knows that there are no specialty beds at the accepting hospital, therefore, the hospital does not have the capacity to care for the patient. The specialist is like a general, when he or she gives the order "yes" or "no," it is followed.

As stated earlier, the transferring physician needs permission to put a responsible physician name on the transfer form. If there is no name, there is no transfer. Remember, if the accepting emergency physician accepts a transfer using his or her name, he or she is now responsible for providing emergent medical care. If his or her specialty consultant has not been contacted prior to transfer and is unavailable, the accepting physician has now become the transferring physician and the hot potato has been passed.

Emotions run high when the hot potato is an infant or child, as you will see in the next chapter.

18

THE LITTLE BUNDLE OF JOY

IT IS COMMONLY KNOWN THAT KIDS are not just small adults. Children often have very different medical needs and often require very different medical care than their parents or other adults. An emergency physician at a community hospital must be equally comfortable caring for infants, children, and adults. A sick infant or child often places extra stress on the emergency medical staff. This is primarily because most young patients present to the emergency department for non-life threatening medical problems. When a very ill young patient does arrive, the tension in the emergency department can be palpable.

There are two main venues where infants and children may receive emergency medical care. Some hospitals are dedicated exclusively to care for infants and children. These children's hospitals or medical centers have extensive pediatric experience, specialty pediatric equipment, and specialist physicians and surgeons who dedicate their medical careers to care for these younger patients. If your child needs an advanced medical or surgical procedure, there is a good chance that the medical staff at a children's hospital has performed the procedure many times before. As stated in previous chapters, experience is the key to an optimum medical result.

One very common invasive procedure that is done on sick patients is intravenous catheter placement for a lab draw or to give medications or fluids. Dedicated pediatric nurses are usually very competent in performing IV placement on infants and children, as these are the only patients that they care for. This type of pediatric experience and clinical skill is most important when it is your baby or child on the other end of the needle.

Caregivers should be aware that there are some hospital emergency departments that have very little experience in caring for pediatric patients. These emergency departments are usually adjacent to, or close to, a pediatric medical center, thus, the emergency physicians and nurses do not routinely care for younger patients. If the emergency medical staff does not feel comfortable caring for your child, you should not feel comfortable either.

Fortunately, most hospital emergency departments are capable and qualified to care for younger patients. Caregivers should be aware that most community hospitals provide medical care to patients of all ages. It is not uncommon to have a one-month-old patient in a room next to an eighty-year-old patient. Most community emergency physicians are capable and experienced in providing medical care to anyone who walks or crawls through the door.

Despite the fact that community hospital emergency departments do not exclusively care for pediatric patients, most are very experienced in caring for these younger patients. As long as your emergency physician and nurse are clinically experienced and comfortable with caring for your child, the medical care should be on par with any pediatric medical center. The only exceptions are pediatric patients who are extremely ill or require an emergency special procedure or intervention. These patients may have to be transferred to the care of a specialist at a pediatric medical center. As stated in a previous chapter, this transfer process can be a frustrating experience.

Caregivers should be aware that providing emergency medical care for pediatric patients, at times, is very challenging. Children have different medical needs and requirements than adults. Their expression of pain or discomfort can be difficult to interpret. The "snap shot" initial evaluation by the emergency physician may leave out important clues that only the caregiver may be able to provide. Was there a fever? Was there a trauma? What changed on the way to the hospital? These are questions that only a caregiver may be able to answer. If you think something is different or abnormal about your child, write it down so that you can better inform your emergency physician.

The doors of an emergency department are always open. This fact is especially important for sick or injured pediatric patients during the evening and at night, when their pediatrician's office is closed. Most pediatricians provide after hours telephone medicine with the help of an answering service. While this service is often helpful for caregivers, it is also a time of high risk. Things can be missed without a physical exam. Most experienced pediatricians recognize the limitations of telephone medical consultation and send their patients to the emergency department if there is cause for concern. The advantage of emergency medicine is that a physician is always available to "lay hands" on the patient.

The emergency physician may notice a concerning rash, a heart murmur, or signs of dehydration. **In this sense, a physical picture of the patient is worth a thousand words**.

Younger patients, older patients, and all those in between, will, at times, need specialized experience or care in dealing with unique medical or social situations.

19
THE LONELY VOICE

ONE OF THE MAIN REASONS that emergency physicians go into the field of emergency medicine is that it offers a significant variety of patients. Among this large pool of patients are people who are mentally or physically compromised. It is the responsibility of the emergency physician to ensure that these patients are well cared for. Most emergency physicians want to do the right thing and respect the wishes of patients and their family members. The emergency physician often also becomes the patient advocate.

Abused Patients

At times, the emergency physician may have to involve social services or state agencies when there is suspected abuse or negligence. This is often the case with child abuse or elder abuse. At times, this can make the emergency physician an unpopular person. Despite this, the emergency physician has a legal responsibility to report certain things to the authorities, and most will not hesitate, as this is part of their job.

Dying Patients

Emergency physicians also have to deal with unpleasant end of life decisions. Many family members do not want their very sick loved ones to die at home or at a nursing home. At the very end of life, when death is imminent, family members often request that these patients be transferred to the hospital. Sometimes the patient's primary care doctor has already signed a paper that has made him or her DNR (do not resuscitate) and DNI (do not intubate). This essentially means that the patient should not be subjected to medications or procedures to restart his or her heart and that he or she should not have a breathing tube placed in the mouth, even if he or she is not breathing.

Some primary care doctors become frustrated when the emergency physician informs them that their DNR/DNI patient has come to the emergency department seeking care. The emergency physician simply wants to follow the wishes of the patient and the family. In most instances, the patient will be admitted into the hospital and placed on CMO (comfort measures only) status. This means the physician can treat pain and make the patient comfortable without heroic medical interventions. Most family members want their loved ones to be comfortable and, at these times, they often look to the emergency department to fulfill that need.

Socially At Risk Patients

Emergency physicians often are one of the few advocates for the homeless and those with mental illness or substance abuse. Very often, these patients slip through the cracks in society and the emergency department is one of the few places that they can turn to for medical care or help. Most caring emergency physicians will obtain a social services consult, may give a meal, or may dispense needed medications that can calm the patient. The emergency department staff may assist in drug or alcohol detoxification placement or with finding a safe place for the patient to stay the night, such as a shelter. These patients may also be plugged into community resources that may be very beneficial for the patient. Emergency physicians often try to set up medical follow up care with their hospital's medical clinic.

These are patients that other physicians may shun. Emergency physicians give them a voice.

20

THE SAFETY NET

THE EMERGENCY DEPARTMENT IS THE ONLY PLACE in the healthcare system where anyone can go for any reason to seek medical care. No appointment is necessary. There are federal laws that mandate that each and every patient that presents to the emergency department be given a medical screening exam. Unlike private medical offices, the doors to the emergency department are always open and patients cannot be turned away. In this regard, the emergency department is truly society's safety net.

Patients need to be aware that there are many people that collectively hold this medical safety net together. When a patient presents to the emergency department, there is usually someone at a desk who will ask for the medical problem. This person often has no medical training and may be a security guard or a volunteer greeter. This is the "pre-triage" phase of your emergency medical care. The triage phase starts when you see a nurse and your chief complaint is taken along with your medical history. Your vital signs should also be obtained at this time.

If you or a loved one is very ill, ask for a nurse immediately when presenting to the emergency department. Because the hospital greeter may not have "medical eyes," they might not be able to see an impending medical catastrophe. If you have been pre-triaged to the waiting room and your symptoms worsen, you should ask for a nurse to assess you. Remember to ask the person taking your medical information of their medical training. After all, you are at a hospital and this is not an unreasonable question.

Most emergency physicians are hospital based. This means that they are employees of the hospital, and they do not personally send out medical bills for the medical care that they provide. In most cases, the emergency physician provides the medical care, and the hospital sends the bill. As these two processes are separate, there is usually no conflict of interest. Most emergency physicians independently provide the emergency medical care that they deem to be appropriate without outside interference. The insured, underinsured, and noninsured patients all receive the same emergency medical care. In other words, patients can expect an equal playing field.

Most emergency physicians will not bother to ask about a patient's insurance status, as this usually has nothing to do with the medical care provided. In an emergency medical situation, the emergency physician orders the appropriate work up and administers the proper medical care. This is the ideal way to practice medicine, as all patients should be treated equally.

There are two main situations where the emergency physician may ask about a patient's insurance status. The first is when the emergency physician is considering prescribing medications or medical equipment for the patient to have when they leave the emergency department. For example, if the emergency physician knows that the patient does not have insurance or has insurance that may limit or deny certain medications, he or she may prescribe a less expensive medication for the patient's medical condition. The medication prescribed may not be the ideal or best medication, but often times it is better than nothing. Prescribing an expensive medication that the patient cannot afford to fill does not help anyone.

The other medical situation where insurance status is important is in the setting of outpatient medical referrals. The emergency physician is responsible for providing emergency medical care and is also responsible for providing appropriate medical referrals for follow up. When a specialist physician is on call, they are responsible for seeing referred patients from the emergency department for follow up. Despite this responsibility, some of these private physicians often decline to see patients who are uninsured or have certain types of insurance that they feel do not adequately reimburse for the medical care provided. This fact is sad but true. Fortunately, most hospitals have medical clinics available for the emergency physician to use for follow up. The emergency physician is very aware that this medical follow up can be critical. If the patient cannot get into a specialist, they often return to the emergency department. Hopefully, at this point in time, their medical condition has not worsened.

Social workers are also often available for emergency department patients. These social workers can often provide assistance with finding funding resources for medications or special medical equipment. They also can be helpful for providing resources for transportation to medical appointments. If you or a loved one has a need for assistance, don't be afraid to ask for a social worker. They often have better knowledge than physicians with regard to the social resources that are available.

21

ROME WAS NOT BUILT IN A DAY

EMERGENCY DEPARTMENT PATIENTS OFTEN EXPECT that their emergency physician will figure out all of their chronic medical mysteries that their primary care doctor and their medical specialists could not figure out over a long period of time. Emergency physicians are not super heroes and do not have any special powers. The one advantage that they do have is access to special hospital equipment. For example, a primary care doctor may arrange for a head CT scan to be done within a few days, where an emergency physician can get one done and read within an hour, if necessary. In general, the emergency department should not be used for primary care issues, as primary care doctors have offices to deal with primary care medical needs. If you feel that your medical complaint is urgent or emergent and cannot wait, the emergency department is your best option.

Patients should be aware that an emergency department visit for a chronic medical problem offers a view of just one day in time. The emergency exam may be limited and the emergency medical follow up may be nonexistent, as most patients with chronic medical complaints are referred back to their primary care doctors. If you are acutely sick or your chronic medical condition acutely worsens, you will probably be admitted into the hospital for further testing and observation. If you are not acutely sick, most emergency physicians will send you home. In this case, an outpatient work up with your primary care doctor will have to suffice.

Some emergency physicians will call the patient's primary care doctor to obtain information on the previous medical work up for a particular medical problem. It doesn't make sense to repeat the same medical tests, as this makes the patient's medical care inefficient and redundant. Many primary care doctors want to know when their patients seek emergency medical care, and it is a good idea to inform them so they can stay in the "medical loop." Patients should be aware that some emergency departments have the capability of e-mailing, faxing, or simply mailing a copy of the patient's emergency department record to the primary care doctor. Patients should ask if their emergency department has this important capability. If the answer is yes, patients are encouraged to request a copy of their emergency department record be sent to their primary care physician. This will keep the primary care doctor informed, and the medical record up-to-date.

Some patient's medical complaints and conditions are very complicated with different medical problems, medication interactions, and variations on progression of disease. An emergency department evaluation may only be of limited use as this is just a snap shot of the patient's medical condition and may not accurately portray the problem. While it is true that emergency physicians can get test results faster, it is also true that your primary care doctor knows you best. For chronic medical problems, the primary care doctor should be the captain of the ship with the emergency physician being the first mate if an emergent medical need arises.

22

MARK YOUR CALENDAR

THE PARTICULAR DAY OF THE WEEK and time that you
present to the emergency department can have a major impact on your emergency department medical care and your
hospital experience. In most emergency departments, the
volume of patients gradually increases during the morning
hours, peaks in the early evening and then declines during
the night. Depending on the time that you arrive, you may
have a short wait, a long wait, or no wait at all. If you have
a non-emergent problem, try to plan ahead and choose the
morning before the emergency department gets too busy.

The day of the week can also be a factor that determines the speed and efficiency of your emergency department care. Monday is statistically the busiest day of the
week, with each successive day having a slightly decreased
volume than the previous day. As the number of patients in
the emergency department increases, there is greater strain
on hospital resources. Patients often present to the emergency department on Monday with problems that have been
neglected over the weekend. Patients should remember to
avoid the emergency department on "Manic Mondays."

The second day of the week to beware of is "Frustrating
Fridays." Patients should know that the efficiency of their

medical care might suffer if they are admitted to the hospital on a Friday. Very often, a patient who is admitted on Friday will be stuck in the hospital until Monday, especially if the patient needs a special procedure or intervention. In other words, the patient may have to wait until Monday to get anything done. On the weekend, there is often limited availability of specialists, radiology equipment, and time slots for special procedures. This fact makes some patients feel as though they are trapped in the hospital. Remember, specialty service availability only matters when you are that special patient that needs it.

If you are admitted into the hospital on a Friday and your medical need is non-life threatening, you will just have to wait for it to be addressed on Monday. If your medical need is life threatening and the emergent medical procedure or intervention is unavailable, you will probably be subjected to the unpleasant transfer process and will be sent to another facility. This will be very frustrating for you and your physician.

Patients should be aware that with emergency medicine, as in life, timing is everything.

23
DON'T HOLD YOUR BREATH

RECOGNIZING THAT A PATIENT'S TIME IS VALUABLE, most emergency departments track the amount of time patients spend in the waiting room. These emergency department wait times are often stored on hospital computer systems. Patients are encouraged to research how their local emergency department tracks and stores wait times. Patients can call the emergency department and get updated on the current emergency department wait time, if that information is available. Some emergency departments post their current wait times on hospital internet web sites. Some technically advanced hospitals provide emergency department applications that can be downloaded by the patient to a personal digital assistant (PDA) or a cell phone. These applications often provide current emergency department wait times and directions to the hospital. Other hospitals use a texting format where the patient simply sends a text message to an advertised number and receives an automated response of the current emergency department wait time. Some emergency departments are using public billboards on roads to advertise their current wait times. Patients should be encouraged to research whether their local emergency department provides these valuable resources, as they allow for advanced planning.

Despite all the best intentions for providing information to the public on emergency department wait times, patients need to realize and understand that emergency department operations are always in a dynamic state of change. It may be slow one minute and then busy the next. Patients also need to realize that advertised wait times are usually based on the patient who has been waiting in the emergency department the longest. The wait times for some patients may be drastically shorter if they have a concerning chief complaint or they do not look well. Wait times are meant to provide patients with information that they can use to choose when and where they will receive their emergency medical care. This type of community relations resource should be encouraged, as most of the time, it will allow patients to manage their expectations.

Patients need to be reminded that the emergency department is unpredictable and despite planning, some patients will wait longer than they expected. So bring a book to the emergency department and remember... **don't hold your breath**.

24

WATCH YOUR BACK

THE EMERGENCY DEPARTMENT CAN BE A BUSY and chaotic place. Many patients often feel very intimidated in these surroundings. In the ideal world, patients would have a full time healthcare advocate to keep an eye out for their best interests. In reality, the patient becomes his or her own healthcare advocate by default. Some patients are lucky enough to have a family member or friend to help ensure that their medical needs are being met.

With regard to emergency medical care, patients and loved ones should be encouraged to ask questions if something does not seem right. In other words, don't be afraid to speak up for yourself if you have a concern or information that you feel is important about your medical care. During the fast pace of emergency medical care, there is always the possibility that something may be overlooked or missed. Medicine is not an exact science and is more appropriately regarded as an art form with many gray areas. You are responsible for painting an accurate and complete medical picture of yourself.

Many different people will come in and out of your room (if you're lucky to be in one). There will be attending physicians, resident physicians, physician assistants, nurses, nurse techs, medical students, physician assistant students, nursing students, EMT students, housekeeping staff and, at times, security officers. Each of these people will provide a service to you or you will provide a service to them. The physicians, physician assistants, nurses, and nurse techs will provide you with your emergency medical care. You, in turn, will be providing the students with their emergency medical learning experience. Because at most hospitals, the physicians, physician assistants, nurses, nurse techs, and students are all wearing scrubs, it can be difficult to determine who is providing medical care and who is learning.

When a new face walks into the room, ask that person about their job. This will allow you to use the emergency medical staff to your advantage and will also allow you to know what you can realistically expect from the face in the room. If the face is a physician, physician assistant, or nurse, direct medical care should be provided and all your medical questions should be appropriately answered. If the face is a nurse tech, various diagnostic tests, such as an EKG or a blood draw, may be performed. The nurse tech is often also available for special requests such as providing a warm blanket, getting food for the patient, assistance with the telephone, or assistance with the bathroom. If the face is a student, most of the time he or she is there to obtain a medical history or to attempt a procedure such as trying to place an intravenous catheter or draw blood. Patients should remember that all physicians and nurses were once students and for emergency medical care this "hands on" learning experience is invaluable.

If you know a student is in the room, allow them the opportunity to learn about your medical condition. Often patients with serious medical problems can provide valuable insight for students eager to learn. If a student wants to attempt a procedure, such as an intravenous catheter placement in your arm, give him or her a chance. You do not have to give him or her chances, but one simple attempt under the direct supervision of the nurse or physician is usually all the student expects and can hope for. The principle for medical procedures is "see one, do one, teach one."

If you are not comfortable with students, let your physician or nurse know. Patients should be aware that by denying this learning experience, they may be limiting the amount of time the physician may be spending in their room. This is because many physicians provide bedside medical education by pointing out clinical exam findings and reviewing medical management principles. If the student is not allowed to be there, the medical education time will be spent in someone else's room. Remember you may shape the future medical care of another patient. This is the same thing that someone you do not know did for you.

Some people who come into your room will be there for non-medical purposes. The house keeping staff and security personnel may come into your room. These faces will make your hospital stay cleaner and safer. As previously stated, it is sometimes difficult to know the role of the face in the room. If you are unsure, simply ask. The answer may surprise you.

Emergency medical care usually represents the unexpected and unfamiliar. At times, the emergency physician may not know or realize the true medical problem. Patients should be aware that the emergency physician does not have to tell them exactly what they have, as some times this is very difficult in a short period of time. Rather, the emergency physician has to know who is too risky to be discharged home. For example, a patient with chest pain may have simple stomach acid reflux or may be having a heart attack. If its reflux, you avoid spicy foods and you're fine. If it's a heart attack and you are sent home, you may die. When there is uncertainty, there are few people who would be willing to take that chance.

Emergency physicians are generally adventurous people, but they are usually not risk takers. For many patients, their admitting diagnosis will be the same as their presenting symptom. The elderly patient who is complaining of chest pain will usually be admitted with a diagnosis of chest pain. There is a broad differential diagnosis of possible causes for this patient's chest pain. Myocardial infarction (heart attack) is on this list and makes this patient's symptom high risk. Prudent emergency physicians always consider the worst-case possibilities and will not make gambles on the health of their patients. Patients and physicians who consciously or subconsciously minimize concerning medical symptoms are like high-stakes gamblers at a casino. **If you gamble too often with money or health, the house always wins**.

Speak up for yourself and remember that silence can be a killer.

25

THE LOOK

EXPERIENCED EMERGENCY PHYSICIANS AND NURSES know "the look." The look of the patient can elicit a very emotional feeling when the patient does not look quite right. It may be something very subtle or it may be very obvious, but some patients may make their healthcare providers feel as though something bad is about to happen. In these situations, it is important for the medical team to have special equipment available. This may include cardiac monitors, external pacemakers, defibrillators, intubation equipment, chest tubes and, at times, physical restraints.

The eyes of the emergency nurse are just as important as the physician's eyes. As the nurse is often the first person to assess a patient medically, they are in the unique position to sound the alarm early if needed. The emergency nurse will call for a physician to come immediately into the room if the patient looks like they need an emergent intervention. This may be a patient that needs a breathing tube or a child that does not look right. It could be a patient that is about to have seizure or a patient that is about to pass out. This may also include de-escalation situations, where the emergency physician is called to the room of an angry patient or family member, where there is the potential for violence.

The speed with which you or your loved one receives emergency medical care is often based on the triage assessment. Sicker patients or patients with concerning chief complaints will be triaged to a room and seen by a physician faster than well appearing patients with non-emergent complaints. Many of these well appearing patients with non-life threatening complaints may be triaged to the waiting room or the fast track area of the emergency department. Most emergency departments have a fast track area staffed by physicians and physician assistants that provide express and efficient medical care.

The look decides where the patient goes and how fast they get there. A sweaty patient with chest pain will be put in a room immediately and will be seen quickly. While a smiling patient, complaining of abdominal pain and eating potato chips, will be triaged to a room and seen at a slower pace. In general, sick children and patients who are not breathing, or who are unresponsive or gushing blood, get seen first. If someone gets triaged to a room ahead of you, be thankful that you are not as sick as him or her.

There are some patients that do not look well despite all tests being normal. At times, these patients may have a serious medical condition that is too early to detect. Examples include an adult patient with an early stroke or a child with bacteria in his or her blood. For these patients that do not look well, most emergency physicians would favor admission. If the patient looks very sick, they probably are.

26

THE GOLDEN HOUR

WITH REGARD TO EMERGENCY TRAUMA CARE, a few minutes can mean the difference between life and death. This first hour of definitive medical care is called the "golden hour." It is usually this first hour where the patient's medical fate is sealed. In general, the faster that medical care is rendered, the better the medical outcome will be.

The old adage that all bleeding stops at sometime is true. In a traumatic situation, you would hope that the bleeding has stopped because of an emergent intervention by the emergency physician or a trauma surgeon. The other way that bleeding stops is when the patient runs out of blood, which is obviously not the ideal outcome.

The golden hour is not just limited to traumatic emergency situations. This first hour of emergent medical care is also very important in situations such as heart attack or stroke, where time is heart muscle or brain tissue. Emergent medical interventions can have a profound impact on a patient's survival and ultimate ability to function. Patients and loved ones need to be aware that not all hospitals have the ability to offer definitive medical care. For patients who arrive at an emergency department that is unable to provide the emergent medical care that is needed, the transfer process will begin. The time that is wasted during the transfer process can lead to disaster.

Patients should be aware of the golden hour principle and the fact that each hospital has their own strengths and weaknesses. If you have time and a particular medical problem arises, be aware that you or your loved one needs to be at a hospital that can offer definitive medical care. The best advice is to research your local hospitals ahead of time to determine their specialty capabilities. In other words, go browsing the "medical shops" before you need to buy. With this knowledge, you will be able to make the most informed and most appropriate decision about where to go when the need arises. Most people do not plan for a medical emergency, although everyone will have one at one time or another.

Most patients will be sick enough to know when they are in the golden hour and most of them will miss it when it is gone.

27

THE DARKEST HOUR

NOT EVERYONE SURVIVES IN AN EMERGENCY medical situation. Some patients die at the scene and in these cases, the paramedics will call medical control and ask the emergency physician for permission to pronounce the patient dead at the scene. This is for situations of traumatic death, death for a presumed long period of time, or for situations where the patient has a known medical condition and has been made DNR/DNI, where the patient and family members have made it clear that they are declining medical care. Patients and family members need to be aware that an unresponsive patient needs a signed "do not resuscitate" or "do not intubate" paper or have a family member present to decline medical care. If there is uncertainty in an extremely ill patient, most emergency physicians will error on the side of life. Every patient should be asked about their end of life wishes because when they need them to be respected, most patients are unable to express them.

If there is a suspicious or untimely death in the emergency department, police will usually already have been called, and they may want forensic evidence. Examples include clothes and other personal effects that may have been on the patient's body. Bullets and wound patterns are often very important to a police investigation. Some deaths are innocent and some are not.

You need to prepare yourself emotionally for the physical sights you may see when visiting a loved one who has died in the emergency department. You should expect tubes to be in many places. There may be a breathing tube in the mouth, intravenous catheters in the arms, chest tubes in the chest wall, or a Foley catheter tube in the bladder. There may also be a large amount of blood, vomit, or stool on the patient. Most emergency physicians prefer to clean the patient prior to viewing by the family, but in some circumstances, this is not possible.

The state medical examiner's office is called for all deaths that occur in the emergency department. Family members should be aware that all tubes, such as intubation tubes and chest tubes, would need to stay in place until the body arrives at the medical examiner's office. As many patients who die in the emergency department have known end-stage medical problems, most patient deaths do not require a state medical examiner autopsy. If the state declines an autopsy, you can request that the hospital pathologist perform one.

Some family members and loved ones find comfort in finding the true cause of a patient's demise. This is particularly true if the patient's death was unexpected, or the patient's medical course was complicated. Some find solace in finding answers. For others, the autopsy process is too upsetting, and these family members may choose to have their loved one remain undisturbed. Be aware that the autopsy process will disfigure the patient's body to a certain extent, but that the pathologist is usually mindful of the future funeral and grieving process and will try to minimize external physical deformities.

For most patients, the hospital is the place where life begins and ends. **Remember with the proper knowledge of the emergency medical system, some patients can survive and avoid the darkest hour.**

28

DON'T BLINK

DURING THE FAST PACE OF EMERGENCY MEDICAL CARE, things can be missed in the blink of an eye. Physical exam findings such as a heart murmur, abnormal pupils, a rash, or a stab wound on the back can be overlooked. Diagnostic findings such as a heart arrhythmia on the cardiac monitor, a critical lab value, or a subtle x-ray abnormality can go unnoticed. Communication between medical providers and patients may cause misunderstandings. A patient may misinterpret a word that the physician may have said. A verbal order from the physician to the nurse may be misheard. A key detail from a concerned parent or a key symptom from a patient may not register with the physician or nurse. One simple oversight during an emergency medical situation can have devastating consequences.

The goal of this book is not to frighten people, but rather to honestly portray the emergency medical system that we all share. Patients should be aware of the pitfalls in the emergency department so that they can do their best to avoid them. There are certain critical points to this text that can have a profound impact on your emergency medical care. This important medical information was specifically placed in bold type for easy reference. These "take home" points are repeated and summarized so that they are not missed.

Most patients who present to the emergency department want a firm diagnosis of what is wrong with them. While this seems like an obvious and appropriate expectation, sometimes it is not so easy, particularly with vague complaints. The emergency physician must recognize symptom patterns, generate a differential diagnosis (a list of possible causes for the patient's medical symptoms), and order the proper tests to confirm the correct diagnosis. If the emergency physician can't give a firm diagnosis, the patient's symptoms must then be risk stratified, and the emergency physician will most likely admit the patient if the symptoms are worrisome enough to be potentially life or limb threatening.

Remember that specialty medical coverage may be limited at some emergency departments. Patients never know when they may become that special patient, so they need to be prepared and have a game plan. Be smart and make yourself aware of the local specialty emergency medical services available. If you have an anatomically specific medical complaint, such as a hand injury, eye injury, or genital injury, call ahead to confirm that the emergency department has a medical specialist available to care for you.

Patients need to be aware of the potential risks associated with shift changes. During this "danger zone" time, patients should pay attention, and request both medical providers (nurse or physician) come to the room together to review the medical care plan. In this way, the two medical providers and the patient will be on the same page and things will not be missed.

Some patients have chronic medical problems, such as psychiatric illness, where there is the potential for frequent exacerbations. These patients and loved ones are encouraged to plan ahead and develop an emergency action plan. This should include seeking emergency medical care at a facility that has in-patient psychiatric beds and where the patient's psychiatrist has privileges. This will make the patient's surroundings familiar and should make the patient feel more comfortable.

Patients are encouraged to strategically speak up and advocate for themselves. You are encouraged to be assertive, but not pesky. When possible, use your medical condition to justify a request. Patients are reminded of the benefit of a re-examination, particularly if you feel something was missed. Understand that things may be missed during the fast pace of emergency medical care. Patients are encouraged to give physicians a second chance, as this is mutually beneficial.

If you do not understand your medical problem or a medical procedure you are about to have, speak up and ask questions until you are comfortable. Patients are encouraged to write questions down so that they are not forgotten. Be careful what you wish for and be aware that making unfounded medical demands can have an adverse effect on your emergency medical care. Patients are reminded to confirm the experience level of their medical care provider, as this is the most important factor.

Physically examining patients is the key to quality medical care. If you or a loved one is sick, have a physician "lay hands" on you or your loved one. Patients and loved ones should be aware that "telephone medicine," where a physician renders medical care over the telephone, can lead to suboptimal medical care. The emergency department is always open, and you can be confident that someone will see you.

When presenting to the emergency department feeling severely ill or injured, you should immediately ask for a nurse to assess you. Patients should be aware that emergency physicians see patients when they are in a room on "their side" of the emergency department. Most emergency physicians do not routinely go to the waiting room or triage area. In reality, the triage nurse decides the speed of your emergency medical care.

Emergency department operations are fluid and dynamic. Things can change from minute to minute. One particularly sick or injured patient can impact the entire emergency department and can cause delays for other patients. By understanding and accepting that the emergency department can be unpredictable, you can better manage your expectations. Patients are encouraged to be patient.

Gambling with your health is not smart. Some patients and some physicians gamble by minimizing physical ailments. Some patients feel inconvenienced by medical symptoms and choose to ignore them. Some physicians may overlook or minimize a patient's symptoms for various reasons. Being conservative with medical care is the best policy. Patients should listen to their bodies and physicians should listen to their patients and objective medical tests. Sometimes, there is only one chance to do the right thing.

During the golden hour, severely ill patients need express and efficient emergency medical care. Patients are encouraged to seek emergency medical care immediately to make the most of their golden hour. By being aware of local hospital resources, such as trauma surgery specialists or advanced cardiac care, patients can initially present to the right place to obtain definitive emergency medical care. The golden hour is most valuable when it is not wasted during transfer to another hospital.

Educate yourself about the emergency medical system. Modern emergency department capabilities and technology allow for many patients who are on "death's door" to be saved. Plan for your medical emergency because it is going to happen. By expecting the unexpected, the patient arrives in the emergency department prepared and empowered.

Good health and good luck.

Surviving the Emergency Room: Patient Notes

ED Arrival Time:_____

Chief Complaint (Main Reason for Visit):_____
_____

Medical Questions:_____
_____

ED Physician or PA:_____ Shift time:_____

ED Nurse:_____ Shift Time:_____

ED Tech:_____ Shift Time:_____

Medical or Surgical Specialist:_____

Abnormal Labs or Radiology Findings: _____
_____

Diagnosis:_____
_____

Treatment:_____
_____

Prognosis:_____
_____

Disposition (home, admit, or transfer):_____

Estimated Time for Leaving ED:_____
_____